I0421130

25 Natural and Effective Anti–Aging Tips, Tricks, Secrets And Techniques

All rights Reserved. No part of this publication or the information in it may be quoted from or reproduced in any form by means such as printing, scanning, photocopying or otherwise without prior written permission of the copyright holder.

Disclaimer and Terms of Use: Effort has been made to ensure that the information in this book is accurate and complete, however, the author and the publisher do not warrant the accuracy of the information, text and graphics contained within the book due to the rapidly changing nature of science, research, known and unknown facts and internet. The Author and the publisher do not hold any responsibility for errors, omissions or contrary interpretation of the subject matter herein. This book is presented solely for motivational and informational purposes only.

Table of Contents

Introduction

Are you looking to live a longer life and that too in good health? Do you want to look younger both at heart and in your looks even when you touch 60 years of age? There are simple lifestyle changes and practices that you should incorporate into your day to day life in order to stay fit, healthy and hearty. Many of the problems in people arise when they are completely stressed out and do not lead a simple life. It is important for you to add calorie reduction as well as exercises into your daily routine like your work in order to sustain a good and healthy living habit. This will make sure that you live long and energetic and enjoy all the good things that life has to offer you.

What Does Anti Aging Mean?

Anti-aging is defined as the delay or retard of an aging process. Your body is made up a number of cells and aging occurs when these cells die. In an infant and a child, the blood cells will be strong and resilient and will also help in the formation of many new cells. Even in your every adulthood, you will find that your blood cells are very active and help in the formation of new cells in your body. But, as you age, the ability of your body to produce new cells starts to diminish and death of the live cells occurs. This is when aging steps in. Aging is a phase of life that nobody wishes ever happens. But, with proper care of your diet, health and skin, you will be able to reverse or delay the aging process in your body by a few years. You need to active and physically fit right from your early adulthood and eat the right foods in order to reduce the aging process of your body. A lot of mental tensions, overload of work and stress in your life will tend to make you age sooner than normal. So, it is important for you to lead a stress free and tension free life to reduce aging problems.

Causes For Aging

Aging is one of the common studies that man has undertaken and aging has been scientifically studied by many biogerontolgists. There are seven scientific causes of aging: cell loss, extra cellular cross links, intracellular junk, mitochondrial mutations, extra cellular junk, nuclear mutations and epimutations and cellular senescence. All these are scientific terms and are out of reach for a common man. There are a few general reasons that can be attributed to aging in people. The iron content in the tap water that you drink every day is one of the main sources of aging. The oxidation of the iron will damage the skin and hence makes it dry and sagging. The free radicals in your body are also one reason why you age faster than normal. These radicals will cause damage to the skin and will also trigger the growth of tumors and cancer cells on the skin. If you are overexposed to the sun, then your skin is an easy victim of damage and you become easily prone to a lot of skin diseases. You will only be able to delay the aging process of your body and to protect your body from aging by eating healthy food and exercising regularly. You need to live a very healthy lifestyle if you do not want to age quickly and to live a younger and longer life.

Make The Change From Within

If you do not want to age quickly and would like to lead a normal and healthy life, then you need to make a few changes to your normal lifestyle to reduce easy aging and to prolong the normal body aging process. One of the most important things that you need to consider in your vision to beat natural aging is to stop bad nutrition intake. You need to get proper nutrition at all times in order to stay fit and healthy. You need to put in that extra bit of effort to eat healthy food everyday and this will ensure that your skin enjoys good health and there are no visible aging signs on your skin.

You also can reduce the effects of the dangerous free radicals in your body by eating the right foods that have more quantities of anti-oxidants. Eating a lot of fruits and vegetables that are brightly colored is one way of doing away with the free radicals in your body that causes aging prematurely. If you do not want to age quickly, then you need to first change your sleeping habits. Sleep deprivation is one of the main causes of aging in people. Nobody has the time to sleep the recommended 8 hours every day. More often than not people sleep for just 5 to 6 hours a day. It is important for you to give your body complete rest for a minimum of seven to eight hours every day so that your body gets restored and rejuvenated for the tough day ahead. You are less likely to fall ill if you have rested your body adequately and your immune system will be performing properly.

There are many people who smoke a lot and there are many people who consume more alcohol. But, smoking and consumption of alcohol is not a good sign as far as aging is concerned. Drinking alcohol is an unnecessary addition of calories to your waistline and excessive drinking of alcohol will result in liver damage. Smoking is one of the main reasons for many people to age quickly. Smoking easily affects your skin and you tend to look aged despite your young age. It is also very harmful for your lungs. So, it is highly important for you to show some restrain to bad habits and use it in moderation if you want to lead a healthy life for long. You have the chance to reverse the clock by providing your body with the daily nourishment that it needs.

Anti-Aging Medicine

Anti –aging medicine has come into existence now and is considered to be the clinical or medical specialty that helps in early detection, prevention, treatment as well as reversal of age related problems. The anti-aging medicine is one of the new and fast growing medical specialty. This Anti-aging medical specialty is a long drawn process as it involves anti-aging diagnostic and treatment practices and are supported by scientific evidence. It is based on the proper processing of the acquired data in order to develop as scientific approach to carry out effective treatment.

Solutions Through Anti Aging Medicines

The anti aging medicine is formulated in such a way that it improves your health and slows down aging by targeting the reasons for premature and poor aging. Hormonal decline is one of the main problems of aging and hormone modulation is a solution that will help in downplaying the hormones that boost aging and also to adjust upwards the hormones that will help in reversing the symptoms of aging. It is highly important to maximize and to optimize nutrition as well as digestion and one of the techniques that is followed in the anti aging medicine process is solution to poor digestion and diet. With the help of a proper diet plan you will be able to age well through proper nutritional cleansing of your body. It will help in reversing the metabolic decline in your body, tissue degeneration as well as to prevent the failing of your immune system. It is also part of the anti aging medical specialty to help you to develop good habits and to get rid of the sedentary lifestyle out of your system. You will need to develop healthy and good habits in order to be youthful and to maintain good body vigor. Another important solution that anti aging medicine offers you is the proper functioning of your organs. With the help of natural restorative therapies, your organ functions will be restored and you can be assured that your organs and the systems will be functioning in the highest possible manner.

Tips And Tricks To Anti-Aging

Reversing aging is one of the golden words that many men and women love to hear these days. If you take a look at the advertisements that appear in magazines and newspapers you will see suggesting you injections or creams or lotions or fat removal surgery or hair dyes and so on to make you look younger than what your age really shows. Anti aging products are the norm these days and most of the people do not like to age with time. Aging is not something that you should be ashamed of, but looking old is not one that everyone will digest. Although there are a lot of anti aging cosmetics and treatments available in the market, you can reduce the aging shown on your face and your body by adopting plenty of natural ways that will slow down the aging process. It is very important for you to feel younger inside as this will help you to look younger as well. The following are the tips, trick and techniques that you can use to stop aging soon.

Reducing The Stress

One of the most powerful reasons for aging is the stress experienced by the person. Studies have found that chronic stress reduces the lifespan of cells and the formation of new cells in our body. So reducing stress is essential to prevent pre-mature aging. The person will get better sleep when the stress level decreases and this prevents the symptoms of aging such as wrinkles under eye bags etc.

- Exercise is the best way to reduce stress

- Spending time with friends and family or with children reduce stress

- Practicing yoga or listening to music are other options to reduce stress

The Sun's rays contain harmful ultraviolet radiations which will create free radicals in the body and increases speed of the process of aging and cause the appearance of wrinkles and black spots or pigmentation of the skin. The UV rays destroy the collagen found in the skin, which is necessary for keeping the shape of the face. Small quantities of the sun's rays improve the production of vitamin D which is necessary for the proper development of bones.

- Use proper clothing while going out in the sun to protect your skin from harmful UV radiation.

- Use sun block with SPF (sun protection factor) 15 or above while going out in the sun

- Avoid sun between 10 a.m. and 4 p.m. do outdoor exercises early in the morning or during late afternoon.

Our body is what we eat. There are many foods that help to combat the aging process in the body. The special nutrients present in these foods help to fight aging. These foods reduce the free radical formation in the body which is the main factor for aging. It has been found that food items that contain antioxidants can stabilize the free radicals produced in our body and prevents cells damages including that of skin cells.

- Include anti-aging foods like Avocados, Walnuts, Berries and Beans in the diet.

- Green tea, red wine and water help to fight –off age related problems.

- Eating green leafy vegetables and deeply colored vegetables and fruits reduces high blood pressure, prevents cancer and heart diseases which are associated with the aging process.

- Dark Chocolate is an excellent food when it comes to fight aging as it contains several healthy chemicals which are necessary for the proper functioning of the body.

Have Sex

Having regular sex is another way to control aging signs. Sex is like good workout. Sex improves your heart rate and improves the blood circulation to different parts of the body. It also helps to burn calories.

- Have more sex to prevent early aging signs.

- Practice different positions so that different muscles get toned.

Ground flax seed, virgin olive oil and fish like salmon are rich sources of these fatty acids. It is better to get these fatty acids from natural sources than using the supplements available in the market.

- These fatty acids help to retain the moisture content of the skin and prevent dryness of the skin which provide a younger looking skin.

Smoking affects our skin and other body organs adversely. Smoking can cause bio-chemical changes in the skin. It destroys the collagen and elastin present in the skin, making the skin to sag and wrinkle. Smoking can prevent the proper blood flow through the blood vessels and slows down cell growth.

- The repetitive facial expression during smoking causes wrinkles

- Smoking makes aging faster through biochemical damages

Stimulate The Brain

To prevent aging, it is necessary to have a vibrant and a sharp brain. Our brain needs stimulation to keep it healthy and active. It is necessary to do brain exercises to have neurological fitness.

- Try to learn a new language

- Play brain games which keeps you engaged and interested

One of the best things to keep your body young and energetic is to exercise. Exercise improves blood supply to the tissues and improves cell growth. It reduces the fat deposits in our body and makes the person feel more energetic. Sweating during exercise expels the harmful wastes from our body.

- Get 30 minutes of moderate exercise 5 times a week reduces the aging process.

- Exercise reduces the risk of cardiovascular diseases and cancer

- Regular aerobic exercises increase the bone density

Good Supplements

If you want to achieve anti- aging easily, you can consider taking supplements of anti-oxidants. Sometimes, we may not be able to include anti-oxidant food items and the necessary nutrients required by our body in our diets. Having a nutrient supplement or anti-oxidant supplement will make things easier for you.

- Supplements should be taken to protect your body

- Consume supplements after consulting your doctor to achieve the best result

Get Good Sleep

Your body needs proper sleep to do the repair works in the body and to generate new cells. The lack of sleep can speed up aging by preventing the natural repairing process of the body. People who sleep less than six hours a night may develop high blood pressure, heart attack and are at greater risk of having a stroke. Your ability to remember things and to concentrate will also decrease.

- People lacking proper sleep are more prone to diseases

- For longevity and for physical health it is necessary to have 8 hours of night sleep.

Oil Bath

Taking an oil bath can reduce aging effect on the skin. Massaging sesame oil on the body before taking a bath will help to improve the blood circulation. The oil also re-hydrates the skin and removes the dead skin, giving the skin a healthy glow. This will make you look younger.

- You can use heated sesame oil to get better effect.

- You can also use virgin coconut oil or olive oil to massage the skin.

Fish oil contains omega-3 fatty acids which are necessary for healthy heart and improving immune system in the body. Your skin will look healthy and hair growth will improve when you are taking fish oil capsules as supplements.

- Look for fish oil supplements which are pesticide free

Cleanse Off The Make-Up

Avoid using more make-up on your face once you are above 40 years of age. The chemicals in your makeup can clog the pores in the skin and prevents the skin from breathing. This will make the skin appear as wrinkled and blemished. Cleanse your face before going to bed and allow the skin to breathe.

- Use cosmetics with natural ingredients

- Remove any make up from the skin as fast as possible

Avoid White Sugar

Processed sugar speeds up aging by binding to collagen in the skin and weakening them. This may lead to sagging of the skin and pre-mature aging.

- Avoiding sugar reduces the excess intake of calories and the person will feel more energetic

Lifestyle Changes

If you are in middle age and you want to reduce the speed of aging, it is necessary to change into a lifestyle that is healthy. Making lifestyle changes even in your middle ages can provide you anti-aging benefits.

- Start having a healthy diet

- Start exercising

- Eat and sleep at the right time

Prevent Illness

Illnesses or diseases are a major cause of aging and they cause the body to age faster. To prevent faster aging, it is necessary to prevent certain illnesses like heart diseases, diabetes, cancer and high blood pressure.

- Avoid the use of fatty foods that can lead to cardiovascular diseases and diabetes.

- Try to control blood pressure with the help of exercise and controlling sodium intake.

- Include more of cancer preventing foods in your diet.

Give A Boost To Your Hair

When you get older your hair start thinning. Giving a boost to your hair make you look younger and gorgeous. There are volumizing shampoos and spray gels which will help you to boost the look of the crown.

- The volumizing sprays and shampoos work like collagen injection and helps provide more thickness to your hair.

- It is necessary to apply the sprays near the root of the hairs to get the best result.

Processed Foods

Due to the changes in our lifestyle in the present days we become overdepedent on processed foods. Processed foods contain various preservatives which are harmful to the body. They contain added sodium, more sugar, more saturated fat and less of fiber. These foods can cause diabetes, cardiovascular diseases and hypertension.

- Include more natural and clean foods with essential nutrients and fiber in the diet.

- Read the sodium and sugar content before using any processed food item.

Avoid Anger

When a person is angry or stressed, the level of Cortisol hormone increases in the body and this will have a negative effect on your body metabolism, heart rate, immune system etc. Higher levels of cortisol increase the mortality.

- Learn to forgive and keep yourself cool to live longer.

- Having a good relationship with people makes you stronger and helps to avoid depression and heart attacks.

Have A Positive Attitude

According to researchers, having a positive attitude towards aging can add seven more years to your life. Find ways to achieve pleasure, even when your age is increasing and try to be young at heart.

- Try to enjoy the learning experiences in life

- Try to have more control in your life and enjoy being able to control it.

There are different anti-aging treatments and therapies which helps to reduce aging in men and women. Botox injections and procedure using ultrasound waves are available to give long lasting results.

- These therapies work by increasing the skin elasticity and uplifting the facial tissues.

- Botox is FDA approved treatment for aging symptoms like crow's feet and the results can last for 9-12 months.

- These therapies are costlier than the natural methods and require the help of a specialist doctor to perform the procedure.

Use A Retinoid

Topical creams containing retinoids repair the damages caused by aging effectively. It has found that retinoids which are derived from vitamin-A increases the p-production of collagen in the skin and improves the cell turnover. Retinoids also improves the blood circulation and keeps the pores open which helps to reduce oil deposition and acne formation. However Retinoids are not recommended for women who are pregnant or breast feeding.

- Prescription- strength retinoids are more effective, hence ask a doctor about the right retinoid containing medicine for your use.

- Follow the directions carefully and apply the cream on the face at night as these creams are sensitive to the sun.

There are different spas and beauty salons which offer cosmetic procedures that help to regenerate the skin. These procedures can slow down the skin changes that cause wrinkles and dull texture.

- There are different types of peeling procedures which helps to bring out a new skin.

- Microdermabrasion is another way of achieving younger looking skin.

Socialize

You need to stay connected with people and this will improve your brain power. Sitting in front of the computer or the TV will make you lethargic.

- When you socialize with people you are relaxed and you are learning new things from them.

Reduce The Volume Of Your Headphones

One of the most important organs which get affected by aging is the ears. So, if you want to have good hearing power start reducing the volume of your headphones when you are listening to music.

- Most of us use headphones to hear the music and loud music can increase your blood pressure, anxiety etc.

- Listen to soothing music at low volume to reduce stress and to keep your ears working for long.

www.ingramcontent.com/pod-product-compliance
Lightning Source LLC
Chambersburg PA
CBHW061932280526
45787CB00004B/1580